Contents

The Stress Fallacy:

Why Everything You Know Is WRONG

By C.K. Murray

Similar works by C.K. Murray:

Confidence Explained: A Quick Guide to the Powerful Effects of the Confident and Open Mind

Vitamin D Explained: The Incredible, Healing Powers of Sunlight

Neuro-Linguistic Programming Explained: Your Definitive Guide to NLP Mastery

High Blood Pressure Explained: Natural, Effective, Drug-Free Treatment for the "Silent Killer"

Deep Sleep: 32 Proven Tips for Deeper, Longer, More Rejuvenating Sleep

Mindfulness Explained: The Mindful Solution to Stress, Depression, and Chronic Unhappiness

Emotional Intelligence Explained: How to Master Emotional Intelligence and Unlock Your True Ability

The Fallacy—Stop Thinking Stress is *Bad*!

Stress will ruin your life. If you don't eliminate stress, you are destined to be miserable. There is no place for stress in your life.

Sound familiar? Whether surfing the Amazon Kindle Store or browsing your local brick and mortar, you've seen them: books by the droves claiming that stress is evil. Guides and testimonials that *vow* to leave you blissfully stress-free as you lounge in a hammock, foot in sand, martini in fingers.

While these books seem nice in theory, they're missing a critical point. Stress isn't some evil force that destroys our lives. In fact, stress is a *necessary* part of our lives. Without it, without *some* degree of physical and psychological pressure, we would cease to exist. Stress forces *adaptation*, on the smallest, most critical cellular level. Scientists call this favorable response to stress, hormesis.

Even so, many of us see stress as negative. No matter who we are or what we do or where we go, we face stress. And sometimes, it may seem like the worst thing in the whole, wide world. Regardless of how many palm trees and clear waters grace our presence…

But does that make it bad? Worse yet, are *you* the one making it bad?

When stress hits, we have a tendency to think certain thoughts. Images pop in our minds, visions of failure and inability. Fears of falling flat on our faces, of being weak and weary, of losing ourselves amid the endless barrage of everyday problems. Sometimes, the stress becomes engrained. And we float, our minds constantly at wander. Instead of enjoying the present moment, we think of what we *don't* have, and what we *don't* experience.

It's easy to think that stress is bad, because by and large, that's what we've been taught. When we imagine stress we might picture a lot of things. A man under pressure at work, with his jugular throbbing and his blood pressure through the roof. Maybe we think of a busy single mom, working two or more jobs, zipping from school or daycare to pick up her kids, to drop them off at this or that, to get back to work for the late shift. Perhaps we envision the world of a kid with sick parents, or a struggling student working 40 hrs a week, or a person who was recently fired, or recently dumped, or recently promoted into a position that allows *zero* time for decompression.

Perhaps stress is the reason we say "fuck it." When things get bad, we do exactly what we have to do—we drink. We drug. We exercise, we have sex, we fight, we get hopelessly lost in our technologies. We eat excessively. We run and run and continue to run from the damn demons of our past, from the freaking problems that never seem to end.

Or maybe we simply lie awake at night, wanting nothing more than to stop thinking of today and worrying about tomorrow.

The way we respond to stress sometimes seems unchangeable. After all, we *are* human, are we not? Every now and again we can change our ways, but part of it is just the way we are… right?

Besides, why in the world should we beat ourselves up for doing something wrong or thinking something wrong? Won't that just… well, won't that just cause *more* stress?

Isn't stress the enemy? Isn't stress what gives us high blood pressure, and heart attacks, and strokes, and a variety of other degenerative and acute illnesses, disorders and conditions?

By golly, why in the world would we *not* want to completely eliminate stress?

Well, that's a great question. But what you have to realize is that stress is neither good nor bad. In fact, it's not the stress that kills you. It isn't the stress that makes your chest tight and your vision bleary and your thoughts hopeless. Stress doesn't do that. Stress doesn't do any of that.

Your *reaction* to stress does that. Now, now, this may seem like a meaningless difference, but the truth of the matter is simple: successful people use stress for good. More importantly, *happy* people use stress for good. Sure, it might be nice to be rich and powerful with everything at your fingertips, but not all people who have 'everything,' have everything.

It's easy to be rich and sad. It's easy to be powerful and depressed. It's not rare for some of the most powerful people to be stressed beyond belief, saddled with responsibility, riddled with drugs, doubts, and questionable morals.

Reacting to stress is about more than just managing it. What we should strive to do is *harness* the power of that stress in a way that is conducive to healthy, prosperous living. It's about understanding that our stress is what we make it.

What matters is how we *consciously* apply our stress. And this all begins with how we perceive it.

Conquer Your Conscience—It's all in the Power of Perception

Have you ever been really nervous about something because you wanted it to go well? And right before that *something* happens, you start to notice just how nervous you really are? Maybe you realize that your heart is fluttering or your armpits are getting sweaty, or your face flushed.

And then what happens?

Well, chances are you start to think negatively about these things. Instead of allowing your body to flow, you try to fight it. You think to yourself *I'm so nervous, I'm so stressed*, and then you begin to doubt. As you think about how nervous you are, you create reasons for why you'll fail. Maybe you tell yourself that you can't handle it. Perhaps the more you think about your physiological response the worse it gets.

You sweat more, your throat gets drier, your head woozier, your pulse quicker.

Come on, not now you think. *Why is this happening now?*

But what about days and weeks and years? Forget certain events that trigger stress—what about the *long-term* stress that never seems to end? The type of low-grade, long-lasting stress that wears you down over time, sometimes without so much as a single conscious thought? The kind that settles in your bones and muscles like heavy screws?

Sound familiar?

If so, you're no exception. Everybody will encounter stress, and everybody will endure such stress in its many forms and functions. Sometimes stress feels like anxiety. Sometimes it feels like excitement, or exhilaration, or adventure. At times, it's the pressure on our bodies from exercise. Sometimes, it feels like a heavy weight or a tight chain; many times, we simply feel helpless.

But what if *feeling* bad is simply due to *thinking* bad?

The important thing to remember is that stress is as much a psychological force as it is a physical one. In fact, there is no point in separating the physical from the psychological. They are intertwined; connected. When you think negatively, your body often reacts negatively. When your body reacts negatively, you often think negatively. The same thing applies for positive responses. All in all, the nature of stress is a cyclical one.

Fortunately, we *create* the cycles.

Which is empowering. This means that if we put in the time and the effort, we can learn to control our bodies and minds. And if we control our bodies and minds, we can control the effects that stress has on us.

But wait.

You might be rubbing your head at this point. After all, there will be times in our lives when no matter how badly we wish to control stress, it will get the better of us. Still, the power is *mostly* ours—if we want it.

In order to understand how to harness stress, it would be wise to understand it more clearly. That is to say, what exactly is stress? Can we even define it?

Stress is a hard term to pin down scientifically because it is largely subjective. It is a term based on our *perception* of events and circumstances, with certain conceptions of the term being positive and others being negative. According to the American Institute of Stress (AIS), the term 'stress' was coined by Hans Selye in 1936, who defined it as "the non-specific response of the body to any demand for change".

As the term made its way into everyday talk, it began to mutate. It took on completely new meanings, ones that often ignored the original definition. By and large, the concept of stress became watered down, representing everything from "the non-specific response" itself, the cause of this "response," and the result of this "response."

This makes sense when we think about how people explain their stress. "I'm so stressed," they might say. "I just have so much work." In this case, the cause of the stress is the work, and the response is the feeling of dread or anxiety associated with the work. Over time, we may begin to link the two so closely that they become indistinguishable.

In the end, Selye had no choice but to delineate between the many confusing usages of the term. Eventually, he drew the line by labeling the stimulus the "stressor" and the response the "stress."

Still, isn't it all part of the same cycle? Chicken or egg—which came first? Does it even matter?

In his seminal 1979 book Stress and the Manager, Dr Karl Albrecht defined four common types of stress. Although Albrecht focused on how stress impacted the business world, his conceptions of stress apply everywhere. Basically, he believed that stress was due to the following stressors: time, anticipation, situations, and encounters—with each of the four types conflating in more ways than one.

Fortunately, *all* these types can be used for good. For the time being, however, let's look at how people *misappropriate* them.

1.   Time:

Everywhere you go, there's somebody telling you how busy they are. "Let me check my schedule," they might say. "I'm just so busy, I just don't have any time." People zip around in their cars, on their phones, rearranging their schedules, changing their itineraries, prioritizing this over that, doing this before that, forgetting this, remembering that, trying so desperately to do *everything* that many times they completely come apart. And sometimes accomplish nothing.

Many people I meet complain about how much *stuff* they have to do. They act as if all these obligations and to-dos are somehow pushed upon them, as if they themselves didn't bring on at least some of this stress—as if it all just fell out of the sky. These people are so neurotically caught up in their frenzied schedules that they don't even have the time to say "hello." Ironically, they're so focused on living life that they fail to ever really experience anything. It's all just a fleeting mess. Sometimes I wonder if they even have time for a bowel movement…

Other people run the opposite end of the spectrum. They're stressed by the fact that they don't have time to do anything. However, it's not as if their schedules are full. Instead of doing what they want to do with the time they have, they sit by and *think* about what they want to do with the time they have. They feel trapped; ineffective. They feel as if the whole world is passing them by…

People who stress as a result of time are the same people who plan too much or plan too little. These are the people who struggle to prioritize, who have no idea what they want or when they want it—so they try to do it all. Or maybe, they give up trying to do any of it. Because they either spread themselves too thin or don't spread themselves at all, these individuals are constantly stressed. Sometimes they don't make enough time in their day; other times, their days are endless, creating an impossible schedule that leaves them exhausted, with no time to recoup.

Sometimes, time is all about work. If you're not working, you're anxious. You feel meaningless, you feel worthless. When it comes to 'vacation time,' you can't unwind. You think you should be doing something else. You get so caught up in work that when work isn't coming your way, you can't enjoy the freedom. You become addicted. Hopelessly, physically, psychologically addicted to the grind.

And the grind is eating you alive.

No matter your addiction, it is always good to take time off. That is, if you can stop thinking about time in the first place…

2.   Anticipation

Another common source of stress is anticipation, or thinking about the future. *I hope I don't mess up this presentation*, we might think. *I swear, if this business meeting doesn't go off without a hitch…* Or maybe we simply worry about being late. *I can't be late, I can't be late.*

What if I miss 'it'? What if I get in trouble? What if I get fired? What if I let everybody down?

What would I do then??

We anticipate things and we also anticipate what can happen if things do and don't align with our expectations. Sometimes we place the locus of control outside of ourselves, meaning that we assume that we are largely powerless. *If I miss this, it's because of so-and-so, and traffic, and the problem with the oven, and my damn alarm not working...*

These individuals will find fault in everything else, even when it is quite possible that they are partly responsible themselves. People with external loci of control believe that they are weak and ineffectual, just a helpless plank of wood caught up in the crazy river.

On the other hand, people with an internal locus of control will assign *themselves* a great deal of power. If something goes bad, it's because of *me. If I mess up, if I fail, if something bad happens—it's all because of me.* These individuals may take their beliefs so far to the extreme, that they will hold themselves accountable even when external factors were the main reason. There could be a fire or a car accident or a family emergency, yet they will still somehow find a way to blame themselves.

I should have anticipated this, they will think. *It's all my fault that I didn't see this coming.*

Anticipatory stress can be associated with specific events or it can be vague and undefined. Many people internalize a sense of dread about the future. They don't know for certain what they're worried about, because by and large they're worried about *everything.* These stressed individuals will practically wait for things to go bad. Their fear of failure is crippling; their inability to visualize a positive occurrence, debilitating.

3.   Situations

Think of a situation that stresses you out. Having your head buried in work with a deadline approaching? Waiting in line when you've got a million other things to do and you're already running late? Having to commute from one spot to the other, praying to your lucky stars that the traffic patterns stay normal? Going to court, moving to a new place, starting a new job, going on a first date?

Chances are, there are plenty of situations that you find scary or uncontrollable. Some are emergencies that spring out of the blue and get your blood pumping. More often than not, though, these situations involve conflict or loss of status. Perhaps you do something embarrassing in front of friends, family or coworkers. Maybe you've made a critical mistake, and now some vulnerable part of you is clearly exposed. Or maybe you've found yourself in a full-fledged fight. Somebody has called you out, somebody has put you or your loved ones in a situation that changes everything. And now you have to choose: fight or flight.

What's it going to be? Are you stressed yet?

4.   Encounters

Encounter stress is like situational stress. In many of our lives, we are forced to deal with certain people on a regular basis. For the most part, we are able to manage interactions of this kind, but there are certainly instances where things can go haywire. Depending upon the day, your mental and physical state, and the states of those you're meeting, things can get… *dicey.*

Dealing with customers, clients, coworkers, and everybody else barking in your ear is sometimes overwhelming. Maybe you just don't like certain people because they're unpredictable. Or maybe you know exactly what they are—and you hate it. Whatever the personality 'defect,' certain people or groups of people will make you feel stressed. This can certainly depend upon your job or occupation, as many doctors and psychiatrists have to deal with people who either feel bad and/or cannot handle their feelings.

Just dealing with people in general can be too much. Sometimes we need 'me' time. It's no surprise then, that many people return home from their 9-5 jobs and want nothing more than to sit on the couch, eat, watch T.V., and go unbothered. Being around so many people is a type of sensory overload. Some people might be more inclined to handling it; others cannot.

When we are stressed about something, that stress often manifests in one of three ways. Stress can be *acute*, *episodic acute*, or *chronic*. In these terms, stress is either coming in at a blast, coming in at waves, or existing over a long period of time at a lower intensity.

Acute stress is the most prevalent form of stress. It floods our brains and bodies in the *here and now*, usually a result of recent past experiences and approaching demands. Although some people have mastered how to harness acute stress, many people find it to be exhausting. Overdoing on short-term stress can lead to psychological distress, muscular issues, bowel problems, and other troubles.

Most of us recognize what causes acute stress. Oftentimes, we can literally list our acute stressors, everything ranging from losing a business opportunity, dealing with a child's blunder, paying a higher-than-expected bill, taking the car to the shop, and so on.

The damage done by crumbling under acute stress is oftentimes transient, failing to compare to the problems caused by long-term stress. Such problems include:

- **Muscular issues** such as tension headaches, back aches, muscle pressure and tendon and ligament problems.

- **Emotional dysfunction** such as anger, irritability, anxiety and depression. Oftentimes these emotions will overlap and make us feel confused as to our true feelings.

- **Stomach, gut and bowel problems** like heartburn, stomach acidity, flatulence, diarrhea, constipation and Irritable Bowel Syndrome (IBS).

- **Temporary Over-Arousal** contributing to increased blood pressure, fast heartbeat, sweaty palms, dizziness, migraines, clammy hands or feet, heart palpitations, shortness of breath and chest pressures and/or pains.

Like acute stress, episodic acute stress can also be very negative if we *allow* it to be. Episodic acute stress makes a person a study in chaos and crisis. These are the individuals that are always flying from one thing to the next, that have thrown themselves full-on into the fire with no escape plan. When things *can* go wrong, they usually do.

Many people who experience recurring episodes of acute stress are over aroused, easily angered, anxious and very tense. Oftentimes, these people are fidgety and distracted, seemingly *incapable* of sitting back and taking a breath. They are abrupt, and may even appear to be hostile, leading to interpersonal relationships that rapidly come undone. In fact, dealing with these types of individuals can become a real burden— making the workplace an especially volatile environment.

The term "Type A" personality is typically used in the literature to describe these individuals. According to psychometrists and cardiologists, individuals suffering from episodic acute stress will display impatience, aggressiveness, excessive competition, and an endless sense of time urgency. They will have a way of rationalizing their hostility at all turns, and are almost always marked by a conspicuous insecurity. Researchers have found that Type A's are much more likely to develop coronary heart disease than "Type B's," their more relaxed counterpart. However, seeming too relaxed may also be an indication of problems, such as depression or detachment.

Those suffering with episodic acute stress may also come across as endlessly worried. They will predict disaster at every turn, constantly focused on the catastrophic, ignoring reason in favor of a maladaptive view of life. To them, life is forever threatening and unforgiving. When things actually go 'right,' it is only because of luck, and the worried individual will instantly begin finding negativity in the next event. More often than not, such individuals are anxious and depressed, and highly inclined to alcohol and drug abuse.

The sufferer of episodic acute stress will experience consistent headaches, migraines, hypertension, chest pain and heart disease. Sadly, their own experience with health problems will only serve to confirm and reinforce their negative outlooks. What they don't realize is that it is their mind itself that is largely responsible for these problems.

While acute stress and episodic acute stress are powerful and in-the-moment, chronic stress is not. This is the low-grade stress that deteriorates people on a daily basis, season after season, year after year. Basically, chronic stress is a form of long-term attrition. It's the stress brought on by poor socioeconomic conditions, disjointed families, and other feelings of entrapment in marriage, career choice, and lifestyle. Chronic stress can even occur among ethnic divides and rivalries, literally rooting itself in the DNA of warring peoples.

Some chronic stresses come from early childhood experiences that sink into the fiber of our beings and destroy us. These experiences may create a belief system that causes persistent stress for the individual. Such individuals may believe that the whole world is out to get them, that they need to 'preserve' their fake identity, that there is no possible way for them to 'be themselves.' When personality or perceptual issues must be reformulated, self-examination becomes integral.

Although chronic stress is destructive, it is also easily forgotten. People recognize acute stress immediately because it's new; they ignore chronic stress because it's familiar, and in many ways, as comfortable as it is painful.

In other words, we can get used to crummy conditions. Even when getting used to these crummy conditions is ultimately bad for us.

In the end, chronic stress is a lethal force. It kills through suicide, violence, heart problems, aneurism and other degenerative conditions like cancer. The final, fatal breakdown is the result of depleted physical and mental resources. It is the summation of many symptoms that are often difficult to treat and may require comprehensive medical and behavioral options.

Still, let us not forget the important lesson. In dealing with all this stress, we *choose* to be diminished or improved by it. Stress can be our friend! If we want it to be…

Despite encounters and situations and anticipation and time constraints, stress has numerous benefits. Complex, dynamic, and never easily defined, stress can be harnessed to improve our lives on a daily basis.

And this all begins with how we perceive it…

The 'Shock' Factor—Ways Stress Jumpstarts the Mind & Body

Quick, think of the last time your heart was really pumping hard and you were sweating. Was it because of intense exercise? Did you feel good, and happy, and pleasantly afloat in that endorphin-filled state? Or was it a 'bad' experience? Were you super nervous or anxious about something? Did your performance suffer *or* improve as a result?

What was your mindset immediately before and immediately after?

The basic thing about stress is that it is an evolutionary part of us. "The stress response is a normal adaptive coping response that evolved over hundreds of millions of years to help our ancestors avoid sticks and get carrots," says Rick Hanson, PhD, a neuropsychologist and author of *Buddha's Brain: The Practical Neuroscience of Happiness, Love, and Wisdom*

According to Hanson, it's all natural. Whether hunting sabre tooth tigers or constantly exposing ourselves to mild or moderate stresses in our modern, frenzied world—it's all the same! Stress is a response, and it's neither good nor bad. It's simply a response to what we put ourselves through.

Now, this doesn't mean that we shouldn't reduce stress in some cases and increase it in others. After all, our bodies are designed to engage stress periodically, followed by long periods of easy rest. However, our bodies are *not* designed to flee predators 24/7, just as they're *not* designed to be on social networks, websites, cellphones, workplaces, and other avenues 24/7. Sensory overload will get you, and it will get you good.

That being said, our bodies aren't designed to lounge in hammocks in the sand for hours on end either. Our bodies and minds demand some level of stress, some level of pressure, to keep us fit and functioning. Think of it this way: you don't want to turn into Jabba the Hutt. But you don't want to shatter like carbonite either.

Like all things in life, living with stress is about living with balance.

Of course, this is much easier said than done. Maintaining balance in your body and mind is like learning to keep the see saw perfect at all times. In many ways, balance isn't so much about even levels, second after second, day after day. It's about knowing when to let things get hectic, and knowing when to sit back and kick up your feet.

We all struggle with this, and it all begins with learning to avoid extremes. Extremity is terrible. There's nothing wrong with going all out in whatever it is you're doing, from *time to time*. What becomes problematic, however, is when you're *always* going all out. Redlining. Putting your body through the cauldron with no end in sight. Exhausting your resources and running your battery to death.

Stress begins in the brain. The brain is what takes us from easygoing to five-alarm tragedy. The amygdala, which processes emotional data, sends a threat message to the hypothalamus, which then tells our sympathetic nervous system to protect us from the impending 'attack.' Our nervous system then jacks up our heart rate, constricts blood vessels and dilates others, slows down the intestines, changes the digestive secretions, and floods the body with cortisol.

When this alarm is always going off, when cortisol is constantly flushing the brain, you can get "hippocampal brain damage," which messes with your sleeping and waking, makes you moody, and kills your memory. Brain fog much?

When it comes to stress, the pituitary gland also plays a huge role. Our pituitary gland controls the majority of the glands in our body, regulating many functions including body temperature, thyroid activity and urine production. The pituitary gland eventually causes the release of cortisol, which increases arterial blood pressure, and takes glucose and fat from body tissues and throws them into the bloodstream—all in an effort to boost energy.

The pituitary gland also gets our thyroid gland working hard, thus speeding up our metabolism, jacking up blood-sugar levels and increasing respiration, heart rate and blood pressure. Basically, our bodies and minds get the wheels rolling. This is neither good nor bad, as the uptick in our bodies can deliver great results in the short term. However, when the wheels are constantly running at full speed, they tend to get chipped, and broken, and then they fall off.

And nobody wants the wheels to fall off. Like your car, you can only take your body and mind to the shop so many times. After a while, you're *totaled.*

One part of the human engine that shouldn't get damaged is the heart. Blood vessels constrict during the stress response, which makes it tough for the heart to pump blood. When the vessels are constricted, your blood pressure is increased. In short time, this worsens inflammation, arterial plaque buildup and 'bad' cholesterol, thus increasing the risk of heart attack.

Another element that floods your system and affects your heart is adrenaline. Now, we've probably all heard of adrenaline. In short bursts, it is highly effective, giving us impressive strength and mental acuity. However, when adrenaline is constantly released, our lives get out of hand. Our heart rate and blood pressure go up, while our gastrointestinal activity goes down, giving us that feeling of 'butterflies' in the stomach. When this happens repeatedly without rest, we start to feel *very* weird.

Ever been so tired that you couldn't go to sleep? Exhausted yet wired? Ever been physically beaten down, but your mind was racing? Ever been mentally exhausted but your body was *amped*? You get the picture…

When this response to stress occurs regularly without the recuperation we, as humans, require, the adrenal glands start to deplete. Over time, we run out of adrenaline and develop "adrenal fatigue." This shows up as physical ineptness, exhaustion, hormone imbalances, skin problems, immune suppression and depression. Basically, it sucks.

Basically, allowing stress to constantly control us is a sucky way to live. It is also quite painful. Especially in our stomachs. When the thyroid prompts the stomach to under or over produce acids, things can get very uncomfortable. Too much stomach acid leads to painful acid reflux known as heartburn, while too little acid causes your stomach to be ineffective. When ineffective, your stomach will struggle to digest food, causing feelings of bloating and inflammation. Even worse, your body will fail to absorb nutrients from your food.

No matter how amazingly nutritious the food is, if you're too stressed… you won't benefit from it.

The primary stress hormone, cortisol, is a big reason why so many things can go wrong during stress. Although some people may applaud stress for keeping them thinner, stress can also make us heavier. Cortisol prepares our bodies for quick energy by triggering our appetites. Cortisol also floods the bloodstream with glucose which gets stored as fat in our body's tissues. Basically, chronic stress makes us want more food, and then stores that food as fat. You might be an exercise junkie, but if you're constantly stressed by other areas of your life—you'll fail to lose that gut. Then, ironically, as a result of failing to lose weight, you'll only get more stressed. Making weight loss even harder…

Unfortunately, weight loss may be the least of our problems. Chronic stress also affects our romantic and reproductive lives. In women, the hormone progesterone is a necessity for fertility. It is also a creating block of cortisol in our adrenal glands. When the body uses large amounts of cortisol, the total amount of progesterone decreases, contributing to both reduced libido and increased risk for infertility. In a sense, stressing excessively about having children may very well be a major reason for the continued inability to have children.

Aside from reproduction, stress also greatly affects the aging process. Telomeres, the tiny protein structures at the tips of chromosomes, serve to preserve genetic information when cells divide. As telomeres get shorter, cells slowly stop dividing. Cells may also become dysfunctional, leading to serious ailments such as Parkinson's or dementia. In the end, chronic stress accelerates the aging process by chomping away at telomeres and increasing the rate of cell loss.

By this point, stress may surely seem like a bad thing. It may appear to be something that is terrible and destructive and totally anti-life. The thing is, it's *not*. That's because stress is perception. Think of it this way:

You might suffer 4 years of chronic stress. Perhaps you're stuck in a crummy job and a crummy relationship and you feel like your life is going nowhere. Maybe you wake up every day pissed and anxious and frustrated and depressed. Perhaps you feel like there is nothing you can do and you want to just *attack* the nearest person who ticks you off.

But then because of all that stress, you start to do certain things. You begin to say 'fuck it,' and you start acting unapologetically. Then you start to open doors. You begin to find that life is changing because you're finally starting to do things the way you want without fear.

Three years later your life has totally turned around. When you look back, you wonder if that previous period of stress was 'bad.' Perhaps it was, perhaps it wasn't. But didn't it lead to a lifestyle that is now 'good.'? So was it bad that it happened? Was it good?

And what about acute stress? What about the kind of stress that gets your adrenaline pumping and your heart thumping? Sometimes it freaks you out, sure, but it's also gotten you to do things that you wouldn't have done otherwise. Maybe acute stress allowed you to come up with a great idea in a short time period. Maybe acute stress enabled you to have a great competition or a great performance or an outstanding job interview.

Remember, having no stress may also predispose us to physical and psychological problems. If you're a compulsive runner and you run extremely hard every day, studies may indicate that you're actually at risk for increased arterial plaque buildup and heart disease—because you're *overworking* your body. However, if you never run a day in your life, and one day decide to get up and go out for a jog—you might have a heart attack and drop dead. If this occurred, doctors may do an autopsy and discover that your body was ill-prepared for exercise. Perhaps they'd say that your veins and arteries were simply weak, not elastic enough. Maybe your heart valves weren't capable of such acute stress, perhaps your muscles were atrophied, and your lungs wilted.

Again, balance is the main factor when it comes to stress. Research has shown that the immune system may benefit from short bursts of stress because they make us healthier and stronger. However, too much will give us a gut, and a higher risk of cardiovascular problems and type 2 diabetes.

Short bursts of stress may also make us more creative. According to Larina Kase, PhD, stress often comes before or coincides with creative breakthroughs. When our minds are calm, we have no reason to change. However, when discomfort hits, we reach a new level of perception that is both stressful and weird. Inspiration, it seems, favors the stressed and weird. Perhaps it's no surprise then that many creative people are not only eccentric but also engage in 'binges' of certain behaviors when creating their works.

Of course, stress is also brought on by exercise. Although exercise is considered 'stressful' because it literally puts pressure on your muscles and organs, this type of pressure can be beneficial. Regular exercise gives us a good feeling caused by released endorphins; not to mention, an increased resilience to stress in general. Exercise has been shown to regulate levels of cortisol to keep us more balanced, more "zen." However, experts also warn that exercise should not be abused. Like anything, too much of it will defeat the purpose.

Recent research has also shown that short-term stress before a medical procedure correlates with a better and quicker recovery. Stress may even suppress the production of estrogen, a major factor in breast cancer development. The power of stress comes from its ability to affect us physically and psychologically. If we can learn to embrace stress on an intermittent basis, we may actually think clearer too.

In fact, studies on rats find that stressful events cause stem cells to create new nerve cells that then boost the rats' cognitive performance several weeks later. Scientists call this "neurogenesis."

Studies also reveal that low levels of stress in childhood help to reduce negative stress responses in adulthood like inflammation and heart issues. Like rats, humans exposed to moderate stress learn and remember new information more effectively. Humans exposed to low or high levels of stress *do not* exhibit the same type of improvement.

In the right doses, strength emboldens the immune system, improves the efficacy of vaccinations, and may even fight certain forms of cancer. Of course, these 'doses' depend on the way we *perceive* the stress.

The take-home message is this: you don't want to be stressed all the time, and you certainly don't want to be stress-free.

Perception is key. Researchers at the University of Wisconsin-Madison surveyed roughly 29,000 people and asked them to rate their level of stress over the past year in terms of how they believed it had influenced their lives. They were asked to rate stress as affecting their daily living just a little, moderately, or a lot. Eight years later, death records were observed to see who had passed.

The study was interesting. The findings revealed that among those who had reported stress as having a major impact on their lives, the risk of death increased by 43%. On the other hand, those that experienced the most stress but perceived it the most positively, were amongst the least likely to die as compared to all other participants in the study.

Another such study echoed these findings. Employees at a financial institution were assessed on their stress mindset before and after watching a series of videos that either presented stress as enhancing or detrimental. Those individuals who viewed the video that showed stress as enhancing later reported improved work performance as well as less psychological complications.

In general, acute stress is considered more likely to have potential benefits. When it becomes chronic, the immune system is more likely to be affected detrimentally. A meta-analysis of 30 years of research supports this.

Still, acute stress and chronic stress are all products of perception. Believing you are stressed makes you stressed. And believing that this is 'bad' may very well make it so. To call stress either good or bad is a dilemma that calls into question personal values, cultural mores, and a variety of medical biases.

So let's not call it bad or good. Let's call it human. Let's call it normal. Let's call it *under our control.*

Forget What You Know… Stress Can *Extend* Your Life!

Take a quick look at the above pictures of Rhesus monkeys. If you were asked to guess which monkey had endured more stress throughout its 27 years of life, you'd probably choose the one pictured in A & B. Right?

Wrong. The monkey in pictures C & D has endured more stress than the monkey to the left, yet you would never know it. The hair is dramatically thicker and healthier, the eyes are alert, the face is still fairly tight, the muscles and tendons still strong and responsive.

The study, first conducted in 1989, has endured for 25 years. Focusing on the stress-response in rhesus monkeys to dietary restrictions, scientists began with monkeys from 7 to 14 years of age. The control group was allowed to eat freely. Meanwhile, the experimental group began eating a diet reduced in calories by 30 percent. Years later, the unrestricted monkeys had shown a risk of disease 2.9 times that of the dietary-restricted group, and 3 times the risk of death.

The stress put on the system by caloric restriction appears to change metabolic pathways in amazing ways. Not only does this forced adaptation strengthen the regulation of cell growth and repair, but it dramatically boosts basic bodily measures like blood pressure and heart rate, and wards of diseases such as cancer, diabetes, and other degenerative conditions.

In short, forcing your body to use resources more wisely has many positive benefits. Although we have always been taught to give our body what it needs, to cover all the food groups and never feel hungry—the research begs to differ. Stress is challenge; stress is adaptation. When stressed, our minds and bodies can learn to adapt.

But only if we *believe* in our power to adapt.

When we are operating on the edge of our comfort zone, we are standing on a precipice. At this point, we have several choices. We can (a) step back and return to a less threatening world. We can (b) take the jump, fall, and fail. Or we can (c), channel our rushing heart, our clamoring nerves, and jump the chasm—reaching a new territory we never knew existed.

If we continue to view the chasm between our current position and the new position as insurmountable, we'll never go anywhere. We'll flounder and fall apart.

But if we view stress as a springboard to get where we want to go, if we understand that stress is neither good nor bad, but instead serves as an *incentive* to live healthier and happier—what is there to lose?

Think of the aforementioned monkey study. The monkeys that were restricted learned to adapt. At first, the lessened diet was tough. The monkeys were undoubtedly hungry and uncomfortable. However, after a while, the monkeys learned not just to live with the stress; they learned to *embrace* it. Because they could no longer eat like the gluttons in the control group, the restricted monkeys learned to place a higher value on food.

Value and happiness have been correlated in many studies. When people have to work harder for something, they see that something as having more meaning, more value. When something is simply handed to us, we don't learn to appreciate it, and in many instances, we are left feeling unfulfilled and unhappy.

The same thing applies to stress. Having pressure, having resistance, having to work against the grain to get something can be good for us. If it's too easy, we haven't really experienced anything, meaning we haven't really *lived*. If it's too hard, we give up before we start.

This may explain why today's materialistic modern cultures report being less happy than the more experience-driven societies of past. Not to mention, more stressed. Think of the stereotype of the hard-working farmer who goes without a lot of the things you and I take for granted. Imagine a man whose hands are always dirty, who rises with the sun, who toils in the fields and raises the animals—a man who has a smile on his wrinkled face, despite his seemingly menial existence.

What makes this guy so content, you ask? Well, it's because he actually understands the value of work; the simple satisfaction of carving his niche, and knowing his place. He literally and figuratively shapes his world—starting with his bare hands.

When other people talk of the farmer, they sometimes laugh. He's a good, wholesome man, they might think, just a little disconnected from the 'real-world.' Over there, in his farm with his pigs and cows, without even a cellphone or internet...

But what if he's not so disconnected from the 'real-world'? What if when the skies open and the rain pours, he smiles? What if when others are hurrying, or scurrying, missing the beauty of a bright blue day, the farmer is out in his shrine; somewhere with buttercups and soft winds, the warm embrace of the sun on his shoulders?

Other people are stacked two atop three, in colonies called cities.

Maybe good ol' Farmer Joe knows something most of us don't. Maybe we should all take a little more time, *just* a little, to enjoy the moment. Now, this is not to say that there aren't stressed people in all walks of life. And this is not to say that just because you like material things, you're going to be less happy. What this does say, however, is that there is a lesson to be learned. We should strive to fill our inner world, not our outer world, with meaning. We should seek value in everything we do, and enjoy it for what it is.

Instead of constantly thinking about accumulating more things, we should take pause to enjoy the things we have. The people we have. The abilities, talents, thoughts, emotions—that we have. If you take your favorite food and eat it every day, it probably won't be that enjoyable after a while. But when you eat your favorite food only a couple times a year, at a nice restaurant, or with a close group of friends in the perfect setting, then you *truly* enjoy it.

Learning to live with less, it seems, is an important element in happy living. By adapting to a more 'stringent' existence, we are both reducing and increasing stress. We increase stress in the short term as we adjust psychologically and physically to getting by. However, we also reduce stress in the *long-term*; chronic stress.

By breaking free from the shackles of consumerism, acquiring more and more 'things' is no longer a priority. It no longer weighs on us.

Many studies show the link between less materialism, less stress, and more happiness. Again, this is not to say that people who have no materials are happy—surely many homeless or impoverished citizens are not happier than middle-class citizens.

But what it does say is this: changing the way we perceive objects and materials can greatly improve our lives. By putting a greater emphasis on immaterial things like love, family, creativity, and nature, we learn to step outside our daily obligations and compulsions. We learn to loosen up and live a little.

Again, studies show that the stressful material-mindset of modern societies is bad for happy living. According to David G. Myers, author of The American Paradox, today's young adults have grown up with more affluence, less happiness and a much greater risk of depression and social pathology.

Furthermore, research shows that couples with high levels of materialism exhibit lower marital quality than couples with lower materialism scores. In general, studies show that materialistic people are less empathetic and social.

Materialism, stress, and unhappiness. Three qualities that characterize the modern generation. Sounds wonderful, doesn't it?

Fortunately, there is a way around it. You don't have to be a guru to change your life. If you can learn to harness stress, you can learn to live healthier and happier.

So let's do it…

8 Life-Changing Strategies— Easy, Powerful, Everyday Things

By this point, you want answers. Basically, you want to control the stress you have. You want to harness it. So how do you harness it?

1. **Morning Exercise**—Yes, we all know that exercise is good. However, exercise is best when done in the morning. Sure, we all get tired of daily activities, and maybe the thought of rising early to exercise may not be the most appealing, but the fact is simple: it's all about habit.

When you get in a habit of waking up early and exercising, you won't even need coffee. Just doing some pushups, getting in some brief cardio is enough. It jumpstarts your body and creates a positive, refreshed mindset that can improve the rest of your day. Moreover, you'll feel really good about yourself for doing so, and are likely to follow up your morning routine with other healthy habits, such as eating well and being more productive at work.

Basically, when you start your day off right, you're setting yourself up for a great day, day after day. Studies show that morning exercisers exercise more regularly and enjoy better sleep. Even more, early exercise jacks your metabolism for the rest of the day, so you are burning calories without even thinking about it.

Exercising early in the morning also gives you a nice endorphin buzz.

The stress of physical activity aligns your mind and body. It even reduces negative thoughts, feelings, and chemicals in your body from the night before!

You'll feel better and be healthier. Need I say more?

2. **Music**—And I'm not talking about necessarily the sounds of waves or something stereotypically meditative and relaxing. In fact, just listening to any music may better prepare you for the reality of a stressing situation.

By listening to the words and sounds of music, your mind is able to channel its emotions more adaptively. You can learn to hone your anger, to see new angles and solutions, to think more clearly and live more freely. Music can lower blood pressure, reduce the stress hormone cortisol, and jolt the brain into new patterns of thought.

It's no surprise, then, that many people use music to stimulate the mind—just take a look around a study hall at any college! Not to mention, music is used to prepare people for physical competitions, to channel stress before important and taxing tasks. Music is a gateway to synchronicity and creativity.

So use music for your benefit, and allow it to enhance any experience you might be stressing over.

3. **Drink Tea**—that's tea, baby. Most people nowadays drink coffee in the morning to get the body and mind going. Unfortunately, many people have a tendency to overdo it, thus experiencing crashes later on. The problem with caffeine heavy coffee is that causes a short-term spike in blood pressure and may cause the hypothalamic-pituitary-

adrenal to into overdrive. In short, coffee may very well contribute to uncontrollable levels of stress.

As an alternative to coffee, green tea is very useful. It has less than half the caffeine of coffee and contains antioxidants and amino acids that enable the nervous system to run smoothly and effectively without needless spikes.

Tea also helps because it allows us to gain a noticeable boost that is not too much—you feel energized but also clear-headed. This is the perfect blend for dealing with an important task that has you stressed.

4.   **Less 'Stuff'**—You want to get rid of stuff. Living with too much stuff not only clutters your physical space but also your mind space. Too much stimuli stresses us needlessly and makes us unhappy.

When there is clutter, we are less likely to focus on what matters, we struggle to relax, we believe that our work is never done, we feel guilty for disorganization, we lose creativity and productivity, and we struggle to complete tasks on time.

By treading lightly we actually feel lighter in spirit. We are better able to enjoy people and face problems. Reducing our 'stuff' means reducing obstacles to success.

Besides, when we force ourselves to clean up, we only leave behind the things we really treasure—meaning we can spend our time stressing about what really matters.

Don't sweat the small stuff. Clean up your act!

5.   **Body/Mind Dualism**—An important thing to remember is that our lives are meant to be enriching. The human creature is not supposed to spend all day sitting in front of a computer or in a cubicle. When your mind is not being taxed, you're going to feel imbalanced. You may know that you're missing 'something,' but not know what. Maybe you simply feel lethargic or the opposite, anxious.

The hardest thing is finding that balance. If you spend most days doing something physical, your mind still needs to be satisfied. If you spend most days draining your mind, your body still needs to be satisfied. It is good to work both mind and body. It is also good to work them in different ways. Filling out business reports all day probably isn't going to satisfy your creative side. Just like lifting weights all days isn't going to satisfy your cardio.

Go for walks, meditate, do vigorous exercise. Write in a diary, take photos, be out in nature—do something that makes you feel good and happy. Remember, a job doesn't have to define you. Continue to pursue your true passions on the side as you pay the bills. Never give up on your dreams, and don't surround yourself with people who look down on them.

Be practical, be mindful, and always be *you*.

6.   *Alter* **Don't Avoid**—Many self-help books will tell you that the best way to "eliminate" stress is to simply avoid it. While this may seem good at first, a deeper analysis reveals otherwise.

When we avoid something, not only do we never learn how to deal with it, but we don't grow. Instead, we sit back on our laurels, never really challenging ourselves in that regard. And what happens if we're forced into a similar situation later on and there *is* no escape? What then?

Instead of trying to avoid all things that stress us out, it's better to tackle these situations or circumstances head-on. If the situation is making us very nervous and anxious, we should take the time to think about it. Don't suppress the thought—face the thought.

Same thing applies to our emotions. It's better to express them through a healthy outlet like creativity, exercise, or work. Bottling them up will only make them explode at a later time.

If something is really stressing us, we should strive to alter it. We can do this by compromising, by being assertive, and by managing our time more effectively. All of these acts will help to change ourselves and the source of our stress.

Don't run away from your problems. Approach them, assess them, and attack them. Be smart, be confident, and be unflinching. Remember, stress is what you make it!

7.   **Sleep**—Tired of hearing this one? Well too bad, because it's actually one of the easiest strategies for harnessing stress. And when done right, it makes the biggest changes. Like all things, sleep is about balance. Too little sleep leaves us feeling like crap or edgy. Too much sleep makes us lethargic and depressed.

Harness your stress so that it's at its lowest by bedtime. Do everything stressful during the day. Get your crazy emotions and thoughts out throughout the waking hours and don't postpone your worries till the last minute, when your head is on the pillow.

This all begins with rituals. Avoid exercise and stimuli like computers or videogames at least an hour before bedtime. Use aromatic oils like lavender and rosemary to ease into rest mode. Eat foods like carbohydrates, bananas, dairy and even turkey to promote sleepiness. Just be sure not to eat too close to bedtime, as heartburn and indigestion can result.

8.   **Biofeedback**—Not sure what this means? Well you should, because it's invaluable. Basically, biofeedback is a technique you can employ to control your body's functions, like your pulse. It allows you to focus on making minute changes in your body by relaxing certain muscle groups and making certain responses automatic.

Biofeedback is great because it's noninvasive, it doesn't require medication, and it gives you a sense of personal sovereignty. Biofeedback can also help with everything from constipation to incontinence to high blood pressure to anxiety and tension. It can even help reduce symptoms during chronic conditions like cancer.

Basically, biofeedback is the most self-reflective way to harness your stress. It allows you to understand your body's innate reactions and to then use them at important times—like when trying to relax, when trying to 'psych up' for major competitions or contests, and in general for improved body control.

Heck, biofeedback can even be used to prolong and intensify sex!

Although biofeedback is typically done alongside specialists with electrodes and other sensory equipment, a lesser form of biofeedback can be done on your own. This form of biofeedback requires a certain level of self-awareness. In short, you must learn to recognize how your body automatically responds to stressful situations. Then you must tell yourself how you would like to respond instead.

If your chest gets tights or your heart rate shoots up, you must learn to focus on loosening those muscles. You must learn to breathe more deeply, to think less about adverse reactions and more about how to pragmatically address the source of these reactions. Again, this involves a series of interrelated techniques such as visualization, muscle relaxation, and controlled breathing.

By meeting with an expert, doing independent research, and practicing again and again, you can learn to master biofeedback. In the end, you will learn to take your nervous, maladaptive reactions to stress and apply them in a way that prepares your body and mind.

This will reduce the temptation to deal with stress negatively through drinking, drugging, and other self-destructive behaviors. Basically, it will make you a self-contained, self-confident individual.

And who doesn't want that??

In the end, stress is what you make it. As much as we may feel completely overwhelmed at times, we must remember that *we* are the ones experiencing it. *We* are the ones who worry, the ones who think bad thoughts, who give up or go hard, who pull our hair out and bite our nails and stay up late and drink our coffee and chug our booze and laugh and cry and call our closest friends because we just don't know *how* we're going to make it…

We are the ones who create our lives. Every day, every second, we can choose to structure our lives in one way or another. Every day, we can choose to be one person or another. Change is an act of will. It starts in the mind, with a simple seed. If we want to change, if we want to put ourselves in the pressure cooker, then we can. If we want to lead a more leisurely life, then we can.

How we think about everything that happens is directly related to how our body and mind reacts. So the next time we are stressed, the next time we think we are going to lose it, we should take a step back.

Stress is not evil by default. It is not a shining angel on our shoulder either. It is what we think it is. If we think it will destroy us, it just might. If we think we can use it to achieve incredible things, we just might.

So don't believe the fallacy. There is no such thing as a "stress-free" life, and there shouldn't be. Life is a lot better with some kick.

The Journey: How I Harnessed Stress and Achieved Sobriety

My own journey with stress began when I was young, with wild dreams and stupid thoughts. Although I was a kid, free of worry and all that supposed shit, I began to wonder. There was a world out there and I was beginning to see it.

But more than anything, I was beginning to *feel* it.

We had a big yard back then, and I'd spend my nights staring up, wondering how and why those points of light continued to stare back.

This was the first time I asked the question. The question that haunts everybody from time to time, some more so than others, some more powerfully than they care to admit.

I was scared in those days, well before I should have been. And it was this fear, this inability to know, that would bring me to the darkness.

If you would have told me that I started using drugs on a daily basis because of stress, I would have laughed. I was barely in my teens, *of course* it wasn't stress. Stress was what middle-aged men with jobs and families experienced. Stress was for the worn and wearied, the people that had things to do every day, that couldn't stop lest their lives actually slip out from under them.

Stress was for adults, and me, in my growing, wondrous form, would not have to worry about that for a very, very long time…

But I did worry, and it was this precise worry that led me to the other end. I hated worrying and I hated caring, and so I knew that if I could numb it all away, everything would be okay. Not great, not bad, nothing remarkable either way—just *okay*.

All I've ever wanted to be was okay, but I didn't know. I didn't know that you could achieve something like that without doing something like this—a needle in the arm, pills down the throat, whatever and whenever up the nose and to the brain.

Blood rushing, eyes wide, the cold gasp of death bringing me from nightmare to reality in fleeting succession.

Stress was the reason I wanted to die. But worse than that, it was my reaction to stress that brought that death so close to me. Some days I welcomed it.

Most days, I told myself I didn't care either way.

Which was true. Because I didn't care—I couldn't. That was the point of drugs, after all…

In no time at all, I was deep beyond deep. I lost things and I forgot things and soon the *only* thing that mattered was the haze. I spent my days drugged and that was that. If I wasn't high, I was done. I couldn't do it.

But as long as I stayed under the influence… then *everything* was gravy.

Only after years did it finally click. Did I finally learn to give up the fight and start accepting that life could get dicey. Only then did I realize that *I* was the one in control if I wanted to be. Drugs were unnecessary.

Stress could only hurt me if I allowed it. It is what you make it, I learned. And if you're doing it right, it *just* might make you.

A Special Note:

Thank you for reading *"The Stress Fallacy."* If you enjoyed reading this book and would like to be included on an email list for when similar content is available, feel free:

SUBSCRIBE

As always, thank you for reading.

And may you continue to live healthily and happily.

Sincerely,

C.K. Murray

1. *Mindfulness Explained: The Mindful Solution to Stress, Depression, and Chronic Unhappiness*

2. *Emotional Intelligence Explained: How to Master Emotional Intelligence and Unlock Your True Ability*

3. *The Confidence Cure: Your Definitive Guide to Overcoming Low Self-Esteem, Learning Self-Love and Living Happily*